D0882132

ABOUT DYSLEXIA

UNRAVELING THE MYTH

BY PRISCILLA L. VAIL

Published by

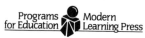

Programs for Education · Modern Learning Press

Book Designed by
Tomasina Walters

10 9 8 7 6 5 4 3 2
ISBN 0-935493-34-4
About Dyslexia. ©1990 by Priscilla L. Vail.

DEDICATION

*To the students
who have been
my teachers.*

CONTENTS

ACKNOWLEDGMENTS

My thanks to the students through whose struggles I have had a window on the glories and perplexities of the dyslexic. I would also like to be a conduit of thanks from those students to the teachers, parents, publishers, researchers, and physicians who work daily for greater understanding, knowledge, therapeutic techniques, and opportunities for dyslexics of all ages.

INTRODUCTION

This book is about dyslexia, a word made from *dys*, meaning trouble with, and *lex*, meaning words. Dyslexia, then, causes trouble with words. This sometimes shows in reading, sometimes in handwriting and spelling, sometimes in listening, sometimes in organizing large amounts of spoken or written information. Because of this, dyslexic students usually have school problems, and may mistakenly be thought unintelligent, lazy, or uncooperative.

Unrecognized dyslexia hurts the self-concept so necessary for leading a productive, joyful life. Therefore, educators, parents, and other adults interested in young people need to understand common patterns of strengths and weaknesses in dyslexic people from early childhood through adulthood. In this guide, we will consider the dyslexic at successive ages and stages starting with pre-school, noticing the effects of dyslexia on school performance and self-esteem.

CHAPTER 1

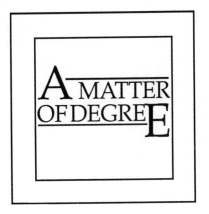

A MATTER OF DEGREE

Dyslexia occurs in roughly 20% of the population, at a 4-1 male-female ratio, among those of average or superior intelligence. It frequently runs in families, so adult readers may recognize themselves, their parents, or their siblings in these pages as well as the children they hope to help by reading this guide.

Dyslexics are often highly gifted in such three-dimensional fields as mathematics, science, music, art, engineering, athletics, or people-to-people skills. However, in two-dimensional symbolic work, dyslexics struggle with reading, handwriting, spelling, and pencil/paper arithmetic.

Dyslexics are often late in learning to talk and, as children and adults, prefer action to words.

Dyslexics frequently reverse or invert letters or numerals, or read and write letters or syllables in confused order. They may have trouble distinguishing *b* from *d* or *p* from *q*, *m* from *w* or *h* from *y*, or 6 from 9. They may read *was* for *saw* or *on* for *no*, or say *callapitter* for *caterpillar*. In later years they may read *unclear* for *nuclear* or *parental* for *prenatal*.

Dyslexics often have trouble telling left from right.

Dyslexics often work skillfully with their hands but make hash of complex verbal intake, output, and organization.

Left-handedness and dyslexia (along with some types of auto-immune disease and migraine) frequently co-exist. They do not cause one another; they are common manifestations of a particular type of brain structure.

Dyslexics are often highly imaginative, creative problem-solvers who have miserable experiences in school, but, given appropriate training, do well in life. Free from pencil/paper academics, they thrive. As Woody Allen might say "There is life after school."

2

Dyslexia is neither mental retardation nor stupidity. It is a different but not lessened way of understanding the world. Some of the famous people said to have been dyslexic are Albert Einstein, Harvey Cushing, Thomas Edison, Woodrow Wilson, Auguste Rodin, and Leonardo da Vinci. In the present time we have such bankers as John Reed, such athletes as Bruce Jenner and Greg Louganis, such actors and actresses as Susan Hampshire, Whoopi Goldberg, Cher, Tom Cruise, such authors as Eileen Simpson, and countless others who are not famous yet (and may never be) who know how to make the world work but have trouble with words.

Dyslexics can learn to compensate but their learning style is permanent. Although this is inconvenient in school years, let us rejoice that no-one "cured" Leonardo da Vinci.

Multi-sensory training, which joins seeing, hearing, saying, and writing in one unified approach to reading and writing our language, helps dyslexics learn the skills needed for survival in our verbal, print-oriented society. Multi-sensory materials may be called VAKT, which stands for *visual*, *auditory*, *kinesthetic*, and *tactile* learning. Such training is appropriate for all learners in all regular classrooms even though it was initially developed for dyslexics.

Dyslexics deserve the understanding help of a society which needs their contributions. As dyslexia itself has different effects, we need to remember that each dyslexic is an individual. That the osprey and the hummingbird both have wings does not make them identical.

Just as intelligence, genius, and talent show in different ways, so dyslexia produces a varied number and degree of abilities and disabilities. It is fitting to link power with problems from the outset, since they are flip sides of the same coin.

3

Margaret Byrd Rawson, psychologist, teacher, and teacher of teachers, and a pioneer in the field, says of dyslexia: "The differences are personal, the diagnosis is clinical, the treatment is educational, the understanding is scientific."

Dyslexia is also a matter of degree, a word with at least five different meanings. Degree can also mean intensity; people can be severely, moderately, or mildly dyslexic.

Degree can also mean an academic certification; it is difficult for many intelligent dyslexics to earn a diploma or a college degree.

Then there is third degree; an inquisition or a burn. Many are the times the dyslexic has been grilled, "What's today's spelling rule?", "What is this word?", "Why can't you learn like the others?", "What's the matter with you...are you dumb, lazy or crazy?". These third degrees burn as deeply as fire, and scar the psyche as surely as the torch does the flesh.

Degree refers to temperature; dyslexics in school have alternately taken the heat or been frozen by misunderstanding.

Finally, degree is a map-maker's tool for marking a place in the world. Literally and figuratively, dyslexics need to know where they stand.

CHAPTER 2

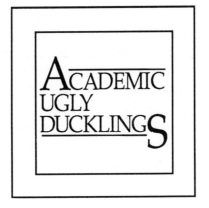

As babies, toddlers, and pre-schoolers display their likes, dislikes, hopes, and fears, each one is a come-to-life Show and Tell. To overlook what children show us about their own learning styles is to ignore the lesson of Hans Christian Anderson (a dyslexic himself) in The Ugly Duckling. In fact, Academic Ugly Ducklings is a good term for many dyslexics.

It is possible to recognize potential learning differences such as dyslexia in young children, and early help may short-circuit trouble. The following children sent important signals.

Bicycle Bill, so-called for his extraordinary large motor skills and balance, mastered a two-wheeler at age 3. He could climb, throw, skate, swim, and row before he was five, but he still held his crayon like an ice pick and hated sitting still; he preferred action to words. Formal schoolwork was to prove painful.

Kindergarten Lucy consistently reversed syllables. She called her favorite foods "bizgetti" and "hang-a-bers," she looked at her mother's "mazagines" and the creature emerging from a cocoon was a "flutter-bye." One day when she looked messy she called herself a "magaruffin." This affectionate, lively chatterbox proved to be a bizarre speller with a severe reading problem.

Joe loved to draw and paint, and could sing on key and pick out simple melodies on the piano when he was only in nursery school. In a seeming paradox, he could draw from memory or copy, but in first grade he couldn't recognize such words as *the, one, Dick, Jane, Spot,* or *Puff.*

Bobby never seemed to listen. No one knows yet whether persistent middle ear infections in early childhood damaged his hearing, or whether he has trouble interpreting spoken language. Both possibilities should have been explored before he got into academic and disciplinary difficulty in 1st and 2nd grades.

3rd grade Gregory loses everything, even himself and his ideas, which come more quickly than his tongue can speak. He has such a poor sense of direction that he sometimes loses his way home. Yet his grasp of numbers and true mathematics is amazing. He is in the lowest language arts group and, because he loses his papers and workbooks, he is failing arithmetic.

These children needed early recognition, and it is not surprising that each one now hates school. But it is never too late to help.

Medical research now shows that the combination of emotional peace and psychological energy opens extra pathways to thinking and learning. Children expand their abilities (and use their strengths to support their weaknesses) when they are in joyful, secure environments. Oddly, the more secure the child feels, the greater his willingness to risk. And without risk, there is no real learning.

When children are in a frightening position or place, they have trouble with memory and with learning new things. A classroom where other children can do what the dyslexic cannot is a place of fear and shame. Therefore, in fairness to the 20% of our population who are dyslexics, we must be aware of the signals they send, and recognize their difficulty as soon as possible. Is this an unfair labeling? On the contrary, it is the doorway to fair practice, because it opens the way to genuine help.

How should we help at school and at home? The first thing we need to do is raise our own levels of consciousness to include an understanding of dyslexic patterns. In schools we

7

should offer pre-school and kindergarten screening to highlight those children who are at risk. This is not to cut them off from school opportunities, but to make sure that school is an opportunity.

We should have multi-sensory methods and materials available in every classroom, for use with any and all children. These materials should be used in reading readiness, and early reading. Teachers can learn to use them quite easily and will be delighted to see their effect on all members of the class.

We need to expose our children to rich language through conversations, questions, and stories. We need to take time for word play and encourage young learners to use words to express their ideas and emotions.

We need to be sure children are aware of their body parts and the two sides of their bodies. Many young children need games to help them remember the difference between left and right.

For children who have trouble organizing themselves in time or in space, we need to show them how to use words as guides. For example, if a student has trouble copying a design, we might say "Tell yourself what is in the design. Three dots, a line to the corner, and then a squiggle." Some children who see the whole do not know how to break that whole into its parts, thus they don't know where to begin, or what should come next.

The Resource List offers further readings and shows where to find specific materials.

Is it harmful to children to highlight them as being at risk? Would it be better to just let them go on their own and see what happens? Let's remember Hans Christian Andersen; to recognize early indications of dyslexia is to distinguish a cygnet from a duck.

8

CHAPTER 3

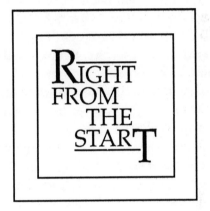

RIGHT
FROM
THE
START

The ready kindergartener is all set to move from learning to love to loving to learn. Most kindergarteners bring hope and happiness over the threshold into the classroom. They are ready to fall in love with both their teacher and their work. How cruel the disappointment and confusion which engulfs the young, unrecognized dyslexic.

Children's opinions of themselves as learners are formed by their first school experiences. Just as the child who can not keep up with the others may build a foundation of anger or sadness, success in the early years breeds zest, flexibility and optimism. With these, almost anything is possible. The child psychologist Erik Erikson says young children believe "I am what I can make work."

First, parents and teachers of dyslexic kindergarteners need to notice what these children do well, and create opportunities for them to show their skills in the classroom as well as at home. Then they need to understand which things are difficult so as to teach *strategies* (much more valuable than answers) for getting around particular problems.

A well-designed, individually administered screening will highlight trouble spots and can be given in half an hour or less, either by a trained teacher or paraprofessional. In developing or evaluating such a test here are some areas to explore.

Copying. Can the child copy geometric designs? If not, does the trouble lie in analyzing the form or in making the pencil obey? Some children, as we mentioned in the previous section, need to be shown how to analyze, others see perfectly well what the form is all about but can't draw the picture accurately. Understanding where the trouble lies is the first step to giving good help.

Letter Naming. Can the child recognize and name letters when they are presented out of alphabetical order?

Word Matching. Can the child find two matching words in a group of four? If not, what are the kinds of mistakes? Do they involve b/d confusion, or trouble with letter order, such as on/no? Seeing the type of error will point to the right kind of help.

Sentence Memory. Can the child repeat, exactly, increasingly difficult sentences you say out loud? If not, are the errors in memory, content, omissions, substitutions, incorrect pronouns, or verb tenses?

Picture Naming. Can the child say the correct label, sometimes called the target word, for what is pictured? If not, are the errors from hesitations, weak vocabulary, incorrect use of labels, naming the function but not the object (fixer-man for plumber), or substitutions within categories (salt for pepper, fruit for vegetables). Word-retrieval problems bother many dyslexics, and they undercut reading skills.

Working with unfamiliar materials and perhaps an unfamiliar person. Is the child active or passive, self-protective or willing to risk?

The patterns which emerge from a combination of exercises such as these highlight those children in need of help. Multi-sensory training in kindergarten and during the summer between K and 1 has often done the trick. The child who learns correct letter formation, letter sounds, and blending has no incorrect habits to unlearn later. Dyslexics need to overlearn these preliminaries. When "I am what I can make work" includes accurate, automatic readiness skills, the kindergarten dyslexic can be in all senses of the phrase "right from the start."

11

CHAPTER 4

KEEPING PROMISES

1ST AND 2ND GRADERS

Intelligent dyslexics whose learning style is not understood are at risk for sad and angry feelings about themselves and school which may remain with them for the rest of their lives. And to tarnish bright promise is really a form of child abuse.

Dyslexic students usually flounder in look-say reading. The, one, Spot, and Puff just don't stick in their visual memories. Katrina de Hirsch, pioneer in dyslexia, says trying to teach sight words to a dyslexic is like trying to make a crisp imprint in very loose sand. Oddly, the child who has trouble remembering sight words may be visually sensitive to artistic or three-dimensional perceptions.

Putting an intelligent dyslexic in a classroom with a look-say reading program can make the child appear *dis*-abled for reading when, in fact, he is *mis*-matched with the materials and method. Conversely, a pure phonics program will produce the appearance of a *dis*-ability in a child who cannot blend sounds into words. In the same way, to put an unready child in a formal academic setting guarantees either failure, discouragement, or rebellion. Such a child may appear *dis*-abled or *dys*-lexic when he simply started too soon. These three examples show us that the learning disabilities can be created as well as inherited.

In order to know what's what, and who's who, teachers and parents need to understand the child's learning style. If individual screening was not given in kindergarten, children who are struggling in 1st or 2nd grade should have diagnostic testing to assess their function in the following areas. (A test such as the Slingerland, listed in the Resource List, does a very nice job.)

The visual system: do they see well, do they see the difference between *b* and *d* or *on* and *no*; do they remember sight words?

14

The auditory system: is their hearing normal, do they hear the difference between *cat* and *cut* or *thrill* and *frill*, can they hear a word such as *cowboy* and repeat it, and then say it again without saying *cow*; can they remember three- or four-part instructions and explanations?

The large and small motor systems: can they manage playground equipment well enough to establish a social place in the group; are their muscles strong enough to do what is asked of them, with both large and small equipment?

The visual-motor system: can they coordinate their eye and pencil; can they remember how to form their letters?

The language system: can they understand the language they hear, can they express their ideas and emotions in words, can they use words and word endings to tell the difference between present, past and future, can they form a question?

The psychological system: are they eager to try, do they expect success or failure, can they focus their attention, and can they make transitions from one kind of activity to another?

The kind of diagnostic testing which produces this information measures *how* the children learn, not *what* they have learned or how smart they are. Accurate diagnosis is the first step to on-target prescription.

Always the adults should be looking for the child's strengths as well as weaknesses, finding where, in Howard Gardner's words, the child is "at promise" as well as "at risk."

1st and 2nd graders need multi-sensory training and when they work on handwriting, spelling, and composition, teachers and parents need to pay special attention to the needs of left-handed students. Southpaws need to learn proper pencil grip and should angle the paper with

15

the lower right hand corner of the paper pointing to the child's belt buckle. This will prevent the awkward, turned-around pencil grip called a hook.

For the unidentified or unaided dyslexic schooling becomes a road block instead of a roadway. In 1st and 2nd grades, the curriculum, not to mention parental hopes, family pride, and student self-concept, focus on learning to read and write. And while appropriate training must be provided to prevent the pain of discouragement, time must also be saved for the exercise of talent. Dyslexics have great promise.

In addition to pencil-paper training, young dyslexics need to hear stories read aloud, preferably by a live adult, but at least on tape. They need chances to pretend, to invent their own personal imagery, and to keep imagination alive. These sources of originality and creativity will nourish their souls, help them over mechanical hurdles, and enable them to keep their promise.

CHAPTER 5

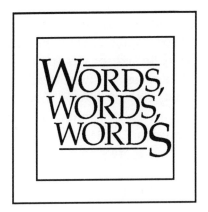

WORDS,
WORDS,
WORDS

"Thirds use words" is how an experienced elementary teacher distinguishes 3rd graders from younger children. At the same time, the curriculum shifts from learning to read to reading to learn.

The competent 3rd grader works with inference as well as with facts, plays with homonyms and riddles, and picks fights or settles disputes with words instead of (or as well as) hands. It is the year for the secret club with ...what else? the secret pass word.

Where does this leave the dyslexic?

In undiagnosed students, those generalized hopes which had kept everyone afloat disappear. Daily evidence contradicts such phrases as: "She'll read when she's ready," "A good summer will fix everything," "If you get 5 Bs I'll buy you a bike," "You could do it if you'd only try harder." These students learn to mistrust themselves: "If I can't do what everybody else can, there's something bad the matter with me."

Students with good ideas but weak mechanical skills ride an emotional yo-yo. The dyslexic with good ideas and bad handwriting can't get his ideas on paper. If he does, they may be illegible. The more rapid or interesting his flow of thoughts, the more likely they are to overload his tired or cramped hand. The result? A mess, an F, or "Copy this entire paper over, correctly please!"

While classmates are polishing their decoding, spelling, word recognition, and other reading and writing skills, using them to discover interesting and important facts and concepts, the dyslexic stumbles over the mechanics he is not ready to use, and yearns for the new information and ideas he can't get from print. Math, likely one of the student's strong points, gets harder if not impossible when word problems appear. When the act of reading is hard, students don't have a lot of energy left over for enjoying it. The dyslexic whose energy is needed for decoding the words "the dragon galloped toward the frightened creatures" has nothing left over for playing with inference.

Who cares why the dragon is galloping when there are 28 more lines to read on the page?

Third grade dyslexics whose learning styles are not understood are caught in a painful gap between the ideas in their heads and the mastery of printed words.

Such students need training to overcome the effects of Specific Language Disability, another name for dyslexia, and must also have opportunities to do what they do well, in the classroom as well as at home. One who draws or builds well might show understanding of social studies by making a diorama or a map instead of writing a report. Another might share insights through body English as well as verbal English, in dance, drama, or pantomime.

These children need exposure to rich vocabulary, and chances to practice using strong, varied words. Language grows through conversation and from hearing interesting words, constructions, and embellishments, not from memorizing word lists.

Thirds use words. The dyslexic at this level needs language training and exposure in order to get his Wordsworth.

CHAPTER 6

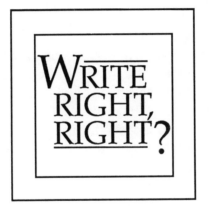

Successful 4th graders are pleased with their own mastery even though they sometimes act silly, as if to ward off the fears and obligations of growing up.

In most schools, 4th graders solidify their earlier reading skills and also increase their verbal powers. They read for content, identifying main ideas, and they can use context or root words to figure out the meaning of new vocabulary. They sort ideas by category, they explain, they defend their ideas, and they write, write, write. To be successful, they need to write right. Topic sentences, simple outlining, accurate vocabulary, and automatic handwriting are their tools.

The dyslexic student may still be struggling to recognize or decode simple words. Many still don't hear the difference between long and short vowels. This means they can't really understand such spelling rules as when to double a consonant, or whether a word is spelled with *ch* or *tch*, *ge* or *dge*.

Many are not ready to organize their written work; they're just beginning to be able to put ideas together on paper. Often, the 4th grade dyslexic's handwriting is cramped, rushed, or sloppy. Developmentally, this is a good time to bring on electronic help. The dyslexic at this age should first learn accurate keyboarding skills. It is vital to establish correct fingering. Hunt and peck will not be good enough for these students who will need to rely on a machine for the final product of their written work. Once keyboard skills jell, the student with access to a computer can learn to compose and edit on a word processor. But the keyboard skills must come first, and be taught separately.

In a well run classroom, 4th graders are generally tolerant of one another, but they are apt to be more forgiving of others than they are of themselves. Dyslexics are often ashamed to admit they need help, and furious with themselves for the botch they make without it.

Two problems which may have seemed minor in earlier years make serious trouble now. First, many dyslexics don't really understand the concept of time. Because time itself is invisible, the only way to understand it is through language. When such words as until, whenever, after, next, or ago don't carry meaning, untrained dyslexics ignore them in conversation and reading, and these students don't develop a grid of time to organize their learning. Because the language of time isn't part of their thinking, they remain in the present tense, cutting themselves off from the ability to sequence. This makes serious trouble in reading comprehension, writing, understanding literature, and history, not to mention planning for long-term assignments. Yet, because the misunderstanding of time is as invisible as the concept itself, the confusion often goes unnoticed and uncorrected.

Second, many dyslexics have trouble finding the words they need as quickly as they need them. This is called word retrieval difficulty. They can't catch what is called the target word. Instead, they ask for "that thing over there;" they describe by function instead of label (the sewing for the needle); they buy time with fillers ("the um, um the, the, um wrench"); or use words that sound nearly right (the McLay/Nearer show for the McNeil/Lehrer show). They forget the names of people, places, things, and dates.

This causes chaos in literature, geography, history, and any subject matter with precise vocabulary. One boy said "I know what 7x8 makes, but when I'm in a hurry I just can't remember the word 56." He does poorly in timed written arithmetic drills although he is a natural mathematical thinker.

Word retrieval problems get worse under pressure for speed or memory, particularly when coupled with writing. In quizzes, test, or exams, familiar words evaporate. Grades go down even though the student says, "...it's on the tip of my tongue."

To help, these students need practice in organizing their vocabulary into categories. This can be done in games and sprint-exercises: "for 30 seconds let's brainstorm all the words we can think of in the category of kitchen equipment ... pot, pan, roaster, oven, timer, spatula, fork, eggbeater, blender" and so forth.

These students need games for pairing words by opposite, synonym, association: hot/cold, damp/muggy, comb/brush. Why? A word stored as half of a pair is twice as easy to retrieve.

These kids need games and exercises showing how words are related to each other by roots and such prefixes as *un* and *re*, or suffixes like *ful* and *able*. Unless they are given this key, many 4th grade dyslexics still think that each word in our language is a separate whole which has to be learned individually. What a wonderful relief it is to discover that if you know the word *think* you can understand, read and spell the word *unthinkable*!

By 4th grade the snowballing effects of undiagnosed or untutored dyslexia are crushing. These students, with average to superior intelligence, suffer outwardly with poor grades, and beneath the surface, with self-doubt. They need training so they can manage those symbols which confuse their ability to think. It is their right to be able to do right, right? They shouldn't be left out, right?

24

CHAPTER 7

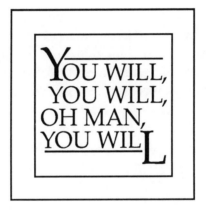

5th and 6th grade dyslexics are stuck with whatever earlier confusions have not been straightened out. The b/d confuser may read *bet* for *debt*. The one who still tangles syllables may read *vacations* for *vaccination* and get a nasty surprise. Some still confuse *were/where/wear* which makes snarls in what they are trying to read. Figures of speech confuse many dyslexics. As Martha said, "I get lost in the shovel."

For these intelligent dyslexics, words which should be landmarks are landmines instead. The language of time continues to make trouble. Who can show me "on the dot," "at two," "around six thirty," or "not until later"?

There are spatial confusions too: the *fifth* is not the same as *five*. Terms of inclusion and exclusion, such as *each*, and *every other*, are necessary for accuracy but unclear to the dyslexic.

Classmates seem to understand the roots and affixes of multi-syllable words. The dyslexic, skilled at taking apart and putting together gears and motors, needs to be shown that a long word such as *manufacture* can be taken apart too. It can be decoded by syllable (man-u-fac-ture); it can also be unlocked by roots: *manu* from the Latin *manus* meaning hand, and *fac* from *facio*, the Latin verb to make.

As mentioned in the previous chapter, developing this kind of word logic lets the student in on the secret. Kids this age love to feel the power of knowing how things work. Literally and metaphorically they love to work the gears.

Understanding roots and affixes helps in spelling and keeps students from making the kind of mistakes which make them look foolish. If he had known *manu* and *manus*, 6th grade Tom wouldn't have written, "I got it from the *man-you-will*." He has heard and spoken the word manual, but he wasn't a frequent reader and the picture of the word didn't stick in his head. He knew it was a book that shows you how to do something. In other words, after seeing the manual, you will be able to assemble the model or work the appliance. So in writing his paper about building a robot he wrote the word as it made sense to him "man-you-will." His paper was returned "Man, you will fail if you don't improve your spelling!"

Here is a Catch-22. Because people are getting better at recognizing dyslexia in young children, some parents and teachers think it is only for little kids, a kind of academic chicken pox; diagnosis, treatment, recovery, immunity. Adults and students alike, then, may be discouraged or even irritated when old problems reappear in new guises. We all need to understand that the underlying learning style is permanent, but its inconveniences can be managed with good training as part of regular classroom teaching.

Particularly as 5th and 6th graders feel the first confusions of adolescence, they need daily evidence that they are okay, valuable people. Exercise and refinement of talent, pursuit of hobbies, focus on strengths--these are vital now and build future strength.

The clumsy, hesitant, embarrassed reader, or the student whose lumpy body still produces awkward penmanship may be drawn to poetry. It is shorter than most prose selections and the rhyme schemes help the reader along, because students this age are both naive and intuitive; they often catch the meaning behind the words. Tom, of *"man-you-will"* fame wrote:

The Cave

Dark, secret, spidery
I go with a lantern
Heart pounding, fearful
Strange noises
What's that smell?
A drop of water
Quick movement in the corner
Farther and farther in I go
Walls closer
What? What now?
Glint! Gold! Treasure!

Providing appropriate help for 5th and 6th grade dyslexics says "You have treasure, and man you will find it!"

CHAPTER 8

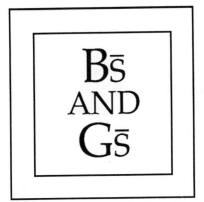

B̄s
AND
Ḡs

Bs and Gs may be short for Boys and Girls, but at 7th and 8th grades, the letters could just as well stand for Blast and Glands. These years of contradictions on the inside and on the outside may be the hardest years of school for the dyslexic.

We need to remember that dyslexia is a matter of degree, and that dyslexics each have individual patterns. Just as all girls named Barbara share a name but are different from each other, one dyslexic (even well-trained) may be an agonizingly slow reader, while another may have trouble with organization. Those with troubles in either the language or the concepts of time and space will have weak reading comprehension. Students whose concepts of time and space are blurred will have trouble with the sequence of daily tasks; moving themselves and their materials to different classrooms, and shifting their thinking from one subject matter to another. Some dyslexics have language difficulties in organizing and remembering what comes in through listening or reading. Other have trouble shaping and focusing what goes out through speaking or writing. In all these cases it is as if a moat separates the intelligent student from academic enjoyment and success.

Students who are slow to digest new words meet increasing pressure in their weakest area. They are expected to understand and use the precise vocabulary of each subject; science, history, math, English, and perhaps even a foreign language.

The 7th or 8th grade student with a mild, moderate, or severe word retrieval problem, which we discussed earlier, will have trouble with classroom discussion, particularly if put on the spot by direct single-correct-answer questions, and will also struggle in written tests or exams. The difference between what this student can do for homework or projects and what comes out on his test papers is an example of the painful inconsistency common to dyslexics at this age.

These also are the years when the misunderstood student can flounder in Developmental Output Failure (DOF), a name first used by Melvin D. Levine, M.D. The gloomy name speaks for itself. It means, a virtual shut-down, first of written output, then of classroom participation. Fear and failure form a partnership which leads to near paralysis.

The roots of DOF often lie in weak handwriting and the difficulty in trying to support an increased flow and complexity of ideas with a lag-behind hand and poor spelling. Such students need consistent training in handwriting in the early years until the skill is automatic, and as mentioned before, they should learn keyboarding first and then word processing.

The student whose dyslexia has been recognized and who is receiving help has a difficult enough time, but the student whose overall intelligence has covered up a mild to moderate dyslexia suddenly can't keep up at this age, and doesn't know why. Disappointed adults may use anger, fear, sarcasm, psychiatry, or bribery if they don't understand the real reason for the downward slide.

7th and 8th grade students long for social acceptance and a respectable place in the pecking order. Being different is dangerous. Dyslexics at this age, who hardly recognize their own faces in the mirror each morning, need structured support from adults they respect in order to respect themselves as different learners.

To Boys and Girls with Blast and Glands, we can offer Bolstering and Gentleness.

CHAPTER 9

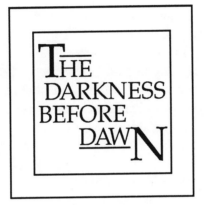

Solid, consistent support is vital in 9th and 10th grades to counteract the temptation to drop out, physically, mentally, or emotionally. These may be the most dangerous years of academic darkness. The idea of quitting school, pumping gas, having a baby, taking drugs, trying crime, or committing suicide may tempt the dyslexic adolescent who can find neither the key to learning nor the key to the exit door.

Pressures to conform, eagerness to be in control, mixed with the inability to control one's own body and emotions, the fact of being a different learner, and the personal uncertainty of adolescence pull the student in contradictory directions.

Parents and teachers need to acknowledge the importance of the dyslexic student's talents by helping to find times and settings for practice of talent and showcases for mastery. When talents are overlooked, the focus of both time and attention turns to what the student cannot do. When negatives steal the spotlight, the talent loses value in the possessor's own eyes, and a life-long source of joy may die.

With pressures for teachers to teach better, for schools to raise standards, and for students to get higher scores on standardized tests, it takes nerve on parents' and teachers' parts to give equal time to talent and to trouble, to remedial work and to what the student already does well.

Ellen's father runs a small business. Her mother is a legal secretary. As a small child, Ellen was slow learning to talk, although she could tie her shoes when she was two, and she was always on the go. She was a weak early reader, a poor speller, and her arithmetic papers were inaccurate and untidy. After listening to an explanation or a set of directions she would smile winningly and say "What?". Her relationship with teachers and other adults in general was one of failure and mutual irritation.

But she had started taking after-school dance lessons at the Community Center, where she was a star pupil. Because her grades were low, her parents threatened from year to year to discontinue her dancing if Ellen didn't improve her schoolwork, but each time Ellen managed to talk them into letting her continue. By 9th grade, her teachers were impatient, her parents were angry, and Ellen herself was sullen and confused.

Then came the class play. She was given the part of "an evil fairy," a minor, non-speaking role. In a costume she had put together with black rags, she took three leaps to center stage and made a series of grimaces as she arched, squatted, threatened, and recoiled, stealing the show.

This was the first time anyone in school had seen a strong side to this weak student. Suddenly her teachers and classmates saw a whole new person: funny, energetic, and capable. The job of getting Ellen through school became important, and thus a joint endeavor. How?

While pencil-and-paper academics, and extended listening continued to be difficult, her teachers found alternative ways for her to show what she had learned. Ellen herself was ready to try harder because she felt accepted. Her teachers and peers thought she was worth saving because they had seen glimpses of a hidden artistry and strength. Her parents were relieved that the world was seeing a positive side to the child they were trying to love. Ellen herself discovered that her dancing was a bridge to other people, and she has gone on to a nationally acclaimed career.

While national fame isn't in every deck of cards, 9th and 10th grade dyslexics need carefully structured adult support to endure those last years of academic darkness until they come into the light of their own accomplishments.

CHAPTER 10

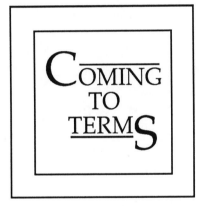

Supported, recognized dyslexics have survived more than 20 academic terms, or semesters, between kindergarten and the end of 10th grade. In 11th and 12th grades the student finally has a chance to make some choices: which electives to take, and what training or education to pursue after high school.

Dean Harriet Sheridan of Brown University says that students who have come to terms with their own learning styles are among the finest candidates for higher education because they know themselves well, they know their own interests, and they can predict what kinds of help they will need. One may need to allow twice as much time for reading assignments as other classmates. Another may need to study in the library, away from the social temptations of dormitory life. Another may need to prepare and polish three or four drafts of any written assignment. Still another may need to have extra time allowed for tests and exams.

Students who have labored to learn what others master quickly often develop a determination and a compassion which boosts their self-acceptance and helps them in their dealings with other people.

For instance, high school students who have survived the system may make successful tutors for younger students, or challenging mentors for others who share a particular interest. Being the helper instead of the helped reinforces the student's sense of self-worth, increasing his willingness to take risks.

In coming to terms with the final academic terms of high school, college-bound dyslexics should tackle the hardest courses they can. This will show college admissions officers their willingness to work on difficult subjects. A lower grade in an "honorable" course makes a better impression than a B+ in a gut.

Most dyslexics need realistic encouragement before they even dare consider the challenge of college, or other forms of higher education. But help must go beyond gathering courage. Student applicants need some specific guidelines for sizing up a program, remembering that evaluation is a two-way process. Here are a few of the questions they should ask:

What am I good at, and which colleges have strong departments in that area?

What is hard for me, and which colleges will allow alternatives, such as waiving the foreign language requirement, or giving extra time allowances?

When I apply, should I submit an extra achievement test score in place of an SAT?

How much extra support will I need, particularly during the first year, and what help does the college offer? It is suicidal to just hope things will work out on their own.

Does the pace of my studying match the rigor of my expectations? It is vital to plan time for friendships, fun, and the exercise of talents. Better a less demanding program and time for social-emotional growth than a prestigious name and an isolation booth.

Parenthetically, it is heartening to see new language arts support programs designed specifically for dyslexics being offered at increasing numbers of schools of engineering and fine arts.

Coming to terms implies both acceptance and endurance. As the dyslexic approaches higher education, coming to terms can also mean arriving at a welcome and welcoming destination.

CHAPTER 11

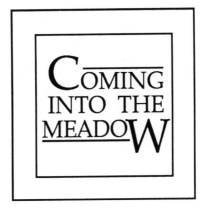

B_y college age and beyond, if the dyslexic's talent has been given time and room to grow, now it can flower. Pride, curiosity, and knowledge build competence and open the doors to opportunity.

Here are some practical suggestions, taken from articles, lectures, and success stories by students themselves, to help the dyslexic make the most of the chance and the challenge of higher education.

Try to get a single room. If it has been hard for you to organize your ideas or equipment, a roommate's or roommates' mess may be a real obstacle to studying, and also to friendship. Conversation, music, and extra visitors during studying time may get you off the track. If single rooms are unavailable, reserve a carrel at the library.

Post a large month-at-a-time calendar over the place where you study. Color-code and mark course dates: class sessions, labs, due dates for term papers, tests, and exams.

Have a separate notebook for each course, keep all notebooks together in one tote-sack or backpack, or on one bookshelf.

Make yourself known to your professor the first session of each course. Explain your interest in the field, your wish to learn well, and mention any special requirements or modifications you anticipate. Don't wait until you are in trouble. If you end up needing no special treatment, nothing is lost.

Get to class early, sit in the front row, organize your materials, take notes and maintain eye contact as much as possible. As soon as class is over, review your notes, underline key statements, and clear up any confusion. Review and be sure you have understood what you have heard before leaving the room.

Be on perpetual lookout for good proofreaders. As Margaret Rawson points out, dyslexics are usually poor spellers who need proofreaders. Dyslexics, like others, usually fall in love with or marry people they have gotten to know. This being the case, good spelling and proof-reading skills should be an important criterion for friendship.

Take time to learn the mysteries of the college's word processing system. It will save your life, but don't try to learn it and use it at the same time. The idea of tape recording lecture notes is a booby trap. Unless you transcribe them nightly, they will be more than any human could listen to in toto.

Make friends with the librarian.

Take the time to plan out your schedule at the start of each semester.

Avoid fatigue and time pressure as much as possible. They revive old ghosts of learning problems. Take temporary setbacks in stride, remembering how much you have accomplished and how many strategies you have for self-help.

Plan time for friends and fun as well as for studying. Follow your interests and try new things. Work remains to be done, but you are free now to choose the field. You have come into the meadow. Take time to look around you, to feel proud, and to set forth.

CHAPTER 12

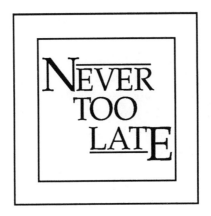

"First comes the carcass" Dick said, gesturing with his left hand, his eyes lit with excitement. "You have to understand where the bones go!" No, Dick is not a butcher. He is a highly skilled cabinet maker talking about making a Hepplewhite dresser. A left-handed man with an artist's sense of proportion and an eye for design, his carving chisel is to wood as Rodin's sculpting chisel was to clay, or Harvey Cushing's surgical scalpel, to brain tissue.

Dick's talk of carcass and ornamentation was a perfect metaphor for understanding, teaching, and encouraging the youthful or adult dyslexic.

First, we must understand the particulars of the situation; we need to know what the dyslexic does easily and what is hard. A program won't work without underlying structure, or skeleton. Next we must plan a course of training which meets the student where he is so we don't go over old ground, and so we are sure we aren't leaving any holes. Once the skeleton of the program is in place, we must find a way of ornamenting it which fits the student's personal interests, taste, and imagination--sometimes expanding on existing interests, at other times reaching out for new ones.

No one wants the plain carcass of a dresser sitting out in the middle of a room. While the carcass establishes proportion and guarantees strength, to be interesting or desirable, the furniture needs its exterior woods, planing, sanding, oil and hardware, which give it form and beauty.

We need to remember this, too. Even trained adult dyslexics, aware of their own tendencies and full of good compensations, who are finally free of schooling and ready to use their talents, may revert to outgrown habits when they are tired or are caught by surprise. Here's an example. Every summer morning, I walk down the street to the store to collect my newspaper. Last summer, in the window there was a sign offering the services of a pro-diver, someone who could retrieve lost moorings or inspect boat bottoms. It took me a month of mornings wondering why anyone would advertise himself as a provider until I understood my error. After coffee I can read, but before breakfast prodivers and providers are all the same to me.

Moderate or undiagnosed adult dyslexics show their stripes by what they choose to do, what they avoid, and by their simple mistakes. They are likely to avoid reading and writing, seeking out other pastimes without realizing why. They make "funny" mistakes, getting files out of alphabetical order, or getting incorrect telephone numbers: 7423 for 7243, or 6932 for 9632.

Misunderstood and undiagnosed dyslexics are also found in jails and prisons, mental health clinics, in menial positions, or in graveyards. Victims of actual or metaphoric suicide, they despise themselves for the symptoms of a condition they do not understand.

It's never too late to help. Dyslexics can learn to read, write and spell. The medical and educational knowledge exists, and proven techniques have done their work. Let each of us, for the good of others and for our own self-interest, reach out to the talented but shackled among us, the dyslexics who have so much to give themselves and their society.

It's never too late.

RESOURCE LIST AND BIBLIOGRAPHY

The following list is brief and representative, and makes no attempt to be comprehensive. The interested reader will, however, find plenty of solid information and will discover ample additional resources.

The Orton Dyslexia Society, 724 York Ave., Baltimore, Md. 21204

Membership in this society is open to all who are interested in the dyslexias. The society is composed of physicians, researchers, educators, parents, and dyslexics themselves. They have a wide bibliography of written materials, and they offer national and regional conferences for all who are interested.

de Hirsch, Katrina. Language and the Developing Child. Baltimore: Orton Dyslexia Society, 1984, Monograph #4. This collection of papers is a gold mine of information about language development in general, and children who are at risk in particular. Written by a legendary figure in the field, it is a scientifically exciting and humanly touching compendium.

Hampshire, Susan. Susan's Story. New York: St. Martin's Press, 1982. This brief, compelling autobiography of the noted actress is a delight to read, and it paints a clear picture.

Rawson, Margaret. The Many Faces of Dyslexia. Baltimore: The Orton Dyslexia Society, 1988, Monograph #5. The papers collected in this volume are scientific, educational, humorous, and above all human. Written by one of the founders of the Orton Dyslexia Society, this volume traces the history of work with dyslexia as well as clinical observations and examples of successful practices.

Vail, Priscilla L. Smart Kids With School Problems: Things to Know and Ways to Help. New York: E.P. Dutton, 1987, NAL Plume paperback, 1989. This book, with case studies, was written for the professional and non-professional reader. It is practical as well as descriptive, and offers information not readily obtainable elsewhere.

ABOUT THE AUTHOR

Priscilla Vail is a nationally recognized authority on dyslexia, learning disabilities and the education of the gifted child. A Learning Specialist and Teacher, she serves on the Advisory Board of The Fisher-Landau Foundation project on The Gifted Learning- Disabled Child and "Gifted Child Monthly." She is the author of "Priscilla's Column" which appears regularly in the Orton Dyslexia Society Newsletter, and is the long-time contributor to numerous newspapers, journals and magazines including the New York Times, Instructor, Independent School and the Journal of Learning Disabilities. Vail's previously published books include in this order: The World of the Gifted Child, Clear and Lively Writing, Gifted, Precocious or Just Plain Smart, and Smart Kids with School Problems. The mother of four grown children, she lives with her husband in Bedford, New York.